AF880773

Pink Tea Leaves

A Collection of Insights from a Breast Cancer Odyssey

Told by Hillary Reed

Written by Trish Thorpe

Copyright

Copyright © 2013 by Fisheye Books:
http://www.fisheyebooks.com

All rights reserved. No part of this publication may be reproduced, stored in a retrieval system, or transmitted, in any form or by any means, electronic, mechanical, photocopying, recording, or otherwise, without the prior written permission of the author.

ISBN 978-0-9853288-4-9
Printed in the United States of America

Disclaimer

Nothing in this book constitutes or is intended as a replacement for medical or legal advice. The authors are not licensed clinicians, therefore you should consult your own doctor before engaging in any activities that result from the information provided here. The publisher and authors disclaim any liabilities for any loss of profit or personal or commercial damages resulting from the use of information contained herein.

Dedication

This book is dedicated to my husband Larry, who has been there every step of the way. And to my loyal chocolate lab "Nurse Chloe."

Life may not be the party we
hoped for, but while we're
here we should dance.

—Anonymous

Table of Contents

From the Author

Hillary and I share a unique connection. She is a former girlfriend of my father's.

We hadn't communicated in thirty years when I reached out to her (via Facebook) in a panic about the direction of my writing "career." She immediately told me "My heart is wide open. Get yourself here as soon as possible."

I accepted her kind offer to let me stay with her and her husband, packed up my life and my car in California, and drove to Colorado. I hadn't seen or talked to her since my late teens, but somehow the elapsed decades didn't seem to matter. We reconnected right away. It's been an extraordinary and positive meeting of the minds and hearts.

After several weeks of living under the same roof, we decided that it made perfect sense to write a book together. At about the same time, Hillary was going through the treatment plan her doctors prescribed for breast cancer.

We talked back and forth about what topic and approach would work best for our collaboration. We both agreed that the world didn't need another clinical, depressing book about breast cancer. So we set our minds to creating something that would capture not only the thoughts and feelings that Hillary was experiencing, but also some of the practical knowledge that she was learning. We also agreed that our book needed to include some of the humor that is so essential to navigating what can sometimes feel like an impossibly difficult illness.

We tried to find a delicate balance between expressions of Hillary's experience and the type of information that would be helpful to other cancer patients. I hope we succeeded.

Trish Thorpe
August 2013

From the Co-author

The idea for a story came to me while sitting in my third chemo session. I had met such interesting and diverse people and I had an idea for a play. The name of the play would be *Bikers,*

Billionaires, and Born-agains. The players, including myself as moderator, would be reclining in four leather chairs with chemo drip stands at their sides. Their stories would evolve and tell of their lives and cancer journeys.

But, I am no writer and was in search of someone who could turn my journaling into an organized book or play. There had been a time in my life when I had been in a relationship with a Hollywood director, and screenwriters and writers were everywhere. But that was some thirty years ago and was a stretch!

And then absolutely out of the blue, Trish Thorpe contacted me. She is the daughter of "my Hollywood director" and is a writer and had just published her memoir. A collaboration was formed and this book was born.

My hope is that it will shed some light on the journey that is breast cancer.

Hillary Reed
August 2013

Introduction

Everyone's cancer journey is unique. And everyone reacts to bad news differently. We get that.

Hopefully we structured this book so that it's as relevant and accessible to as many people as possible.

The chapters are organized in the same sequence that Hillary's treatment was completed. Depending on your own diagnosis, the sequence of events might be different.

Throughout this book, you'll find "call-outs" (prefaced with a small tea leaf and framed by a boxed outline) for practical information that Hillary discovered throughout her journey. We thought it would be helpful for you to read what she learned.

We chose the title *Pink Tea Leaves* for a specific reason. When she was a little girl, Hillary read tea leaves with her great aunt and remembers being fascinated by the random stories that could be told from studying sediments at the bottom of a tea cup. As her cancer odyssey progressed, we settled on tea leaf reading as an appropriate metaphor for the unpredictability of the path that she was traveling.

Also as you're reading, please know that we purposely used a large font (fourteen point) for readers whose eyesight has been compromised.

Finally and thankfully, there's a vast and wonderful selection of books available today to help breast cancer patients feel as medically educated as possible about the choices they face. This is not one of those books. It's not about drugs, doctors, and treatment choices. Instead, it's about women helping women.

Pink Tea Leaves offers the kind of "this was my experience" information that can only come from someone who is navigating the same maze as you. We wanted to share the type of information that women sometimes share with each other over a cup of coffee or tea.

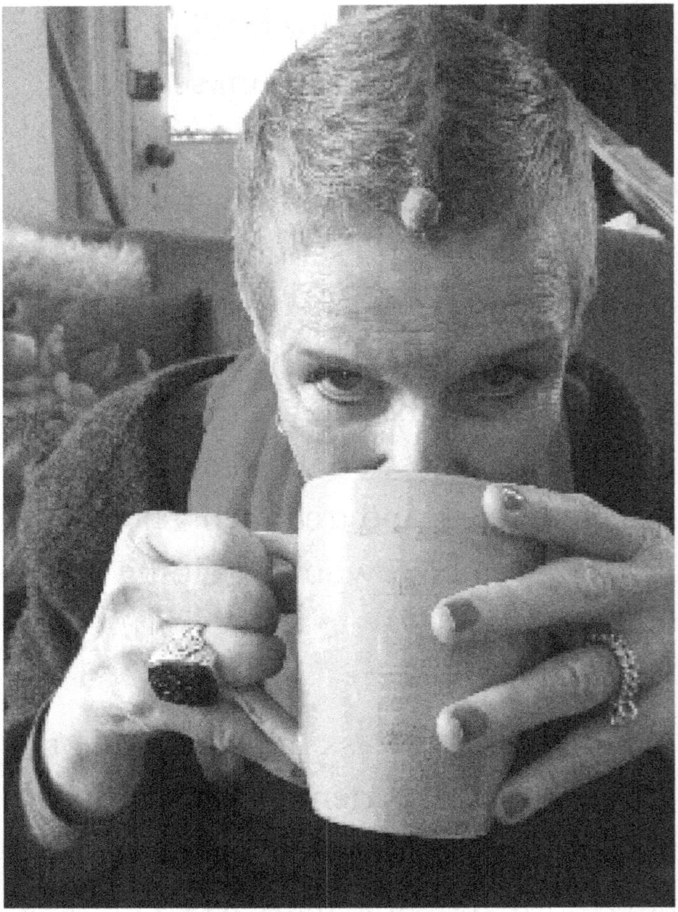

Hillary's Christmas mohawk

I. Diagnosis

"Women are like tea bags. They don't know how strong they are until they get into hot water."

—Eleanor Roosevelt

As I have aged, my body has changed on a daily basis. There is always some new sag or wrinkle to be studied or ignored. I've always prided myself on being healthy, active, and fit.

For months, I'd been noticing that my right nipple had changed. It was kind of retracted. So my right breast looked a little odd to me.

I searched for a bump or a lump almost daily, but because I was feeling for a round mass and not a flat mass, I never did detect it with my fingers. I finally attributed the change to aging and gravity. So did my hubby.

> *Pay close attention to breast shape changes. If you notice that something is different, consult a licensed doctor right away. Don't assume that it's "normal."*

Wrong.

*

I've had annual mammograms faithfully for over twenty years and nothing had ever shown up. When I was diagnosed, the only changes that the radiologist could initially detect were some new calcifications (they show up as white sparkles on the screen). These are quite common in women with dense breasts but because it was new for me, the radiologist scheduled an ultrasound to be sure.

The radiologist read my ultrasound, determined that all was okay, and told me to check back in six months. I went home and didn't dwell on it.

The next morning I got a call from the radiologist saying that he'd been unable to sleep the night before because he felt like something was not right with my ultrasound results. He ordered another one.

As the implications of a second ultrasound began to sink in, I felt a panicked, dreaded fear, but also a certain relief that I was not waiting another six months.

I called my daughter, Karen, and told her what was happening and she met me at the clinic. We sat together silently, staring at the office fish tank, trying not to think the unthinkable. Finally I was called into a room.

This time I had a woman radiologist. She spent a great deal of time doing the ultrasound—much more time than the first radiologist had spent. I watched her face as she clicked on different markers on the screen.

I realized I was in a very serious situation. The screen showed a ten-centimeter mass, shaped kind of like a Band-Aid. It was very deep, and the flat shape explained why I never detected it. She said it looked very suspicious and ordered a biopsy. She told me that I needed to make an appointment with an oncologist.

As I walked out of the exam room, I was close to tears and was trying hard to control my emotions and fear. Looking back, it probably would have been a good time to let it all go and have a good long cry, but that's not my nature.

I walked out into the waiting area. My daughter took one look at my face and knew immediately. She gave me a hug, and we walked out of the doctor's office in silence.

It was as if we'd entered a dream. Everything was in slow motion and looked like it was far away. I felt like I was in the twilight zone.

Mammogram images don't always trigger the proper (or any) alarms.

When we got down to the lobby, we sat down to breathe through the shock. This was all so unexpected and random. I was trying to figure out how to tell others, especially my son, Chris, and my best friend, soul mate, and husband, Larry.

> *The type of breast cancer that you have and its stage at diagnosis determines your treatment plan. Your doctor will be very specific about what will work best for your situation.*

The next days were filled with doctors and planning. Life had changed in an instant. I learned that the tumor had probably been growing inside my body for seven years, and my mammograms never detected it because of its shape.

How could this body of mine that I had taken such good care of ambush me like this? Somehow I thought I was different. I was in shock.

*

I was diagnosed with invasive ductal carcinoma, the most common type of breast cancer.

My oncologist was very thorough in her explanation of my cancer. She told me that, in one sense, I was very lucky because although I had stage three invasive ductal carcinoma, I was also "triple positive." She explained "triple positive" meant that because my particular cancer was fed by estrogen and progesterone *and* I was HER2-positive (usually signifies that likelihood of disease recurrence is high), I would be taking the drug Herceptin, as part of my treatment plan.

I understood from her explanation that I would be on Herceptin for a year. Since Herceptin has been shown to dramatically reduce the risk of recurrence, it signified a very hopeful part of my treatment. I was happy to have that weapon in my arsenal.

In addition to Herceptin, my oncologist explained that I would be on an estrogen blocker for ten years. She also told me that I was to start chemo as soon as my port was installed.

A port is a catheter device that is surgically placed in your upper arm or chest area. The port is used to receive the chemo drugs that are delivered into your bloodstream.

> *I found that Glad's Press'n Seal product worked really well for protecting areas of my body from moisture when showering.*

If you don't want a port, your other option is a Peripherally Inserted Central Catheter (PICC) line. The PICC line is placed in a vein in your upper arm. The exposed valve tubing must be protected from moisture when showering.

A port is considered superior to a PICC line because, theoretically, it's much easier to protect from moisture and bacteria. You can shower like you normally would because the port itself is underneath your skin.

My oncologist told me that I would have six rounds of chemo occurring every three weeks (four and a half months total) and then I would have a mastectomy. Then she told me that as soon as I healed from the mastectomy surgery, I would begin radiation treatment. And after radiation, I could have reconstructive surgery if that's what I wanted.

My next meeting was with the surgeon who would install my port and also perform the mastectomy. My son, Chris, went with me.

My breast cancer surgeon was very attractive, witty, confident, and smart. She was, however, very abrupt and direct when describing my options for treatment. Half of the treatment options that were available to other women were crossed off my list immediately, due to the stage of my cancer.

When Chris asked her about my prognosis, she responded by saying that it was not in her hands and would give no prediction.

The gravity of my illness was becoming clear.

My surgeon installed my port and I was ready for chemo that next day.

II. Chemotherapy

[Alice arrives at the mad tea party.]

Alice: *I'm lost. Could you help me?*
Mad Hatter: *Do you care for tea?*
Alice: *"Have a cup of tea," indeed! Well I'm sorry, but I just haven't the time!*
March Hare: *If you don't care for tea, you could at least make polite conversation!*

- Lewis Carroll
"Alice in Wonderland"

My first day of chemo, I checked in at the front desk and was led to a room with four leather reclining chairs. The room was very sterile-looking. It was painted a cold gray, had a wall of windows to the north, and was kept very cool. Not exactly a cozy environment. But there were blankets and pillows that you could request and bottled water and a basket of crackers and treats.

Each chair had a stand next to it that was holding a bag of fluid. Only two other people were in the room with me that day. A man and a woman. They looked like they were together. They were both so tough and scary-looking (to me) that, to tell you the truth, I probably would have walked across the street to avoid them in any other situation.

> *Wear comfortable clothes and bring a sweater, a book, and/or a smart phone with you to chemo treatments.*

The woman had a chemo drip attached to her arm. She was wearing a pirate scarf on her head and had tattoos covering her huge arms and swollen ankles. The man next to her, whom I later learned was her husband, was wearing a full set of leather biker gear and a matching pirate scarf on his head, was missing teeth, and like his wife, was covered in tattoos. He had a heavy beard that was catching the crumbs of the Ritz Bits he was devouring.

I couldn't help thinking to myself: "Whoa. Where *am* I?"

I decided to keep my eyes down and stay to myself. The nurse came into the room and started my chemo drip.

The drip takes about five hours, so there's plenty of time to think or read or sleep or eavesdrop (my favorite hobby!).

After I got settled, I finally introduced myself to the bikers and they did the same. Their names were Earl and Bet. They were from the eastern plains of Colorado, and this was Bet's last chemo treatment. I learned that they made the long drive into the city on Earl's Harley for every treatment. He was a motorcycle mechanic, and she worked in a gas station in the middle of nowhere.

They told me they had an especially hurtful encounter with another chemo patient during their previous visit. The chemo patient they were talking about, I later found out, was a notable socialite. She had started her chemo three weeks earlier, and in her defense, she was probably feeling terribly scared and out of control the day she met the bikers. No doubt, being cordial to strangers wasn't a priority.

I learned that she had snubbed the bikers that day by adamantly and loudly requesting to be moved to a private room so she could avoid "those people."

As I listened to the bikers talk about how hurt and angry they were, I realized that I had done the exact same thing to them, only in a much quieter way.

It was at that point I realized it was time for me to open my heart and learn who these people really were under that tough exterior. We had a good, long conversation and later exchanged phone numbers. When Bet's treatment finished, they left to start their long journey home on the Harley.

Later that week, I got a phone call from Earl. Bet had died of an aneurysm. It was a fluke, nothing related to her cancer, but Earl was there for her as she passed away.

I think of Bet often and am thankful to have spent time with her. She was a good person, and so was Earl.

*

On my second trip to chemo, I met the socialite who had so offended my new biker friends. Her name was Lucy.

> *You will meet all kinds of people during your chemotherapy treatments – many of whom you probably wouldn't normally hang out with.*

I learned that Lucy only shopped in Paris, only wore cashmere scarves, had a vast collection of huge sunglasses, wore lots of make-up, and had a thick southern accent. She was the wittiest, most wickedly engaging and intelligent woman I had ever met. She loved to laugh and tell stories, but I can see how she intimidated the bikers.

I love her and we became fast friends. But if we had met at some social event instead of chemo, no doubt we would have blown air kisses and complimented each other's hairdos, never knowing a real thing about each other.

*

I had another encounter during chemo with someone whose spiritual beliefs were very different from mine—a born-again Christian. Her name was

Mary, and she sat next to me during my third round of chemo. She was nice, very talkative, and she told me that she was the leader of a Christian women's group and had just completed the study of the Book of Job.

Cancer had certainly shaken my belief system and faith in just about every way, and as I listened to Mary talk, I was thinking about my own belief system. I felt obliged to tell her that I was an agnostic, leaning toward atheism, especially after encountering cancer and feeling like I had nowhere to turn. I told her that even my inner strength felt vulnerable. She was calm and prayerful as she listened and invited me to the next women's group.

A few days later, I told Lucy, the socialite, about my encounter with the "born-again" and the fact that I was feeling like I'd lost my faith. Lucy didn't confirm my skepticism, but instead told me her own story of faith and being led to study the Book of Job.

She told me that when her cancer odyssey began, she, too, had some religious doubts, but her faith had been restored to her in a dream. She told me that when she awoke from her dream, she went to open the Bible that her mother had given to her as a little girl. The Bible, miraculously, opened to the Book of Job.

Well, my faith had new energy after hearing Lucy's story, and I felt an urge to explore the Book of Job. Job's story of redemption seemed particularly relevant to me at this stage of my life, as did his pondering about why the righteous suffer.

Every day presents me with another chance to explore my beliefs and search for my own truths about life. Despite its side effects, chemo does enable downtime for you to explore life's purpose. It also provides extraordinary dreams for you to interpret and ponder.

I believe that all of us rely on some sort of magic or superficial exterior to get through tough times. Whether it's a hard-core, unapproachable appearance (bikers), using money to buy your way out (billionaires), or putting it all in "God's hands" (born-agains), it's all the same.

> *Cancer survival is a combination of head and heart.*

I think the power and strength to fight cancer comes from deep down in each of our spirits, no matter who we are.

*

As I was going through chemo (and beyond), there were some questions I wish I had known the answers to. I have included examples throughout the book.

What happens if the chemicals going into my port leak onto my skin?

After my first chemo treatment, I noticed that my left chest area was red and swollen where my port had been installed. The redness and swelling was getting more severe as the days progressed. It was now late March, and I had been diagnosed in February.

Even though it was late Friday afternoon, I thought I'd better call my doctor to see if I should be concerned. When I described my symptoms, my doctor was immediately alarmed and told me to go to the emergency room.

When the emergency room doctors examined me, they determined that I had an infection that needed treatment immediately. I was quickly admitted to the hospital.

I assumed that my port would be removed that evening and I would be able to go home. But, unfortunately, I was wrong.

I learned that doctors aren't normally scheduled for surgery on weekends. So I remained in my hospital room, port intact, fever escalating, until my family threatened to sue the hospital. April 1st . . . Fool's Day! (Never get sick on a Friday!)

By late Sunday morning, the situation had become dire. I was getting worse by the hour. My husband sat by my side and held my hand. My son and his father went off in one direction of the hospital to find a solution. My mild-mannered, calm brother-in-law (who is a doctor) went off in another direction of the hospital to also hopefully find a solution.

After several heated conversations with various hospital administrators, they all ended up in the same place—the office of the hospital's arbitrator for lawsuit prevention.

My family members explained that they were afraid for my life and that the on-staff doctors were doing nothing to address the situation.

The arbitrator listened intently and then made some phone calls to schedule an emergency surgery.

I looked at the surgeon's face who finally arrived to examine me. He looked visibly shaken as he studied my chest area. I was immediately prepped and wheeled to surgery to remove my port.

After surgery, I remained in the hospital for two weeks while the wound healed where the port had been.

> *Watch your port site carefully. Look for any redness to develop. If it does, call your doctor right away because it may be a sign of infection.*

Initially, the wound got larger and blistered and looked like I'd been horribly burned. Eventually, though, the blisters went away, the wound healed, and I was finally able to go home.

After the ordeal was over and I was back home, I realized that it was a chemical spill on my skin (from a leaking port) that had caused the infection. I wish I had known that, as I was lying in the hospital – it would have definitely made me feel less crazy.

*

Will the chemo make the hair all over my body fall out?

Probably around the same time that the hair on your head starts falling out, your eyebrows and eyelashes will most likely fall out too. Once your eyebrows and eyelashes are gone, consider it a great opportunity to experiment with makeup.

For eyelashes, try using a soft, dark eyeliner pencil to dot in a line where lashes normally grow. To do this, first use a white pencil to highlight the lower lid above the lash line. Then dot in "lashes" with a soft eye pencil (black, violet, or dark brown) on the top and bottom lid.

For eyebrows, I found that powder and a soft flat brush work best to draw natural-looking brows. Start at the end of your eyebrow that is closest to your nose and draw outward. Try to picture the way that your natural brow grows and the shape of your arch. Continue filling in bald spots until your eyebrows are completely grown back.

Don't be alarmed if your lashes fall out twice. Mine did. You should also know that when your lashes do come in, your eyelids will itch like crazy!

Chemo side effects don't necessarily have to be emotionally self-defeating. There are definitely ways to add color and character to each and every body change. Try to make this a creative adventure. You might discover parts of yourself that you weren't aware of.

The hair in your nose also falls out. You have a constant drip because there's no nose hair to catch anything. Carry a tissue at ALL times.

The good news: no more hair growth in unwanted places! No more worries about waxing the hair on your upper lip or chin. And no more shaving your legs or underarms. And definitely no more Brazilian bikini waxes.

All hair *will* grow back a few months after chemo ends. However, the color and texture might change. Straight hair could come in curly and blonde hair could grow back darker.

*

What about fingernails and toenails?

If your fingernails and toenails don't actually fall off, they will most likely become very loose and discolored. They get very brittle and then disconnect from your body except at the nail bed.

I painted my nails with dark-colored polish to cover the discoloration. Dark gray, black, navy blue, and deep purple were my favorites.

I also treated myself to a lot of manicures and pedicures. I experimented with bright colors and patterns too. At one point, I had royal blue and turquoise on every other toe. I think that was my favorite!

Your nails *will* eventually grow back just as strong and clear as they were before chemo. But it takes about a year or longer.

*

Any eyesight changes?

My eyesight was 20/20 before chemo. Now I'm not really sure what it is. I do know that I can hardly read and that my night vision is completely gone. I'm hoping this is temporary. Not sure. I've heard it takes a few years to return to where it was before chemo.

Or maybe the timing of my poor eyesight is just a coincidence. Maybe it's just my body (and eyes) aging and having a harder time adjusting to new focal points.

*

Will my hearing be affected?

I feel like my ability to hear clearly also went down a notch after chemo. My neighbors were the first to point out that my whole house was vibrating from the TV and stereo being turned up so loud. They told me that my car sounded like a boom box.

Again, I have been told that hearing loss may or may not be permanent. There is a lot of "wait and see" on this journey.

*

What about my appetite?

I was lucky and did not suffer from nausea as many women do. However, I had very little appetite and was so tired that I slept almost all day the first week. Even though you're groggy, be sure to drink lots of water so that you don't get dehydrated and require IV fluids.

I do remember my taste buds being different during the first week after a chemo treatment. Things I normally loved tasted like metal or worse. My advice: eat only what tastes good to you! This will all pass.

*

Will my personality change?

I noticed that my social filter went AWOL during and shortly after chemo, so you might want to pre-apologize for anything you say—even to your family and closest friends.

Somehow chemo drugs affect your ability to hold back from saying things that you normally wouldn't. All of the things that you've ever wanted to know or say, but were afraid or too polite to ask or state, seem to lose their "off-limits" status.

Also, it's not unusual to have a trucker mouth at this point in your journey. I swore a lot!

You won't remember much of anything, so there's no need to worry about your lack of filter. It's very freeing, but no doubt annoying to others. My hubby and friends were always good, though, about telling me if I began a story that I had already told.

*

Will chemo affect my sleep?

You might have wild dreams. I did. After my first treatment, I dreamt that little red and sparkling white fighters were inside my body on some kind of reconnaissance mission (scoping out my cancer cells?).

I remember seeing them hovering all over the inside of my body. They reminded me of the figures in some of my grandson's computer games: small, powerful, and heavily armed.

Then during my second round of chemo, I had similar dreams, but this time, the same little figures weren't hovering. Instead they were flying and diving. There were lots of explosions. It looked like what I imagine a battlefield looks like (killing cancer cells?).

My dreams during the next round of chemo were calmer. I remember an indigo-colored dragon's eye that reappeared night after night. The eye would slowly open and look around as if making sure there were no more enemies (cancer cells!) that needed to be conquered.

*

What are my options for headwear after my hair falls out?

Before chemo, my hair was very thick and curly and red and long. I knew it would probably fall out and I didn't want to watch it fall out in large clumps. I started having daily conversations with myself about what to do with my hair.

Should I shave it all off? Should I buy a wig? What style? What color? What would I look like with a mohawk? Should I wear a hat? A scarf? What should I do? I decided to go with my gut.

> *Wear scarves instead of wigs. They're way less expensive, enable more fashion options, and can be removed when your scalp gets overheated without shocking anyone.*

A trip to the hairdresser and a shot of whiskey later, there I was, bald as a baby. Now what? Wig or scarf?

Since wigs can be scratchy, I decided to wear scarves instead, and save the wig for formal occasions. I discovered that scarves can be much more fun and much more comfortable.

For formal occasions, the wig I chose was a bob style. I learned that if you buy a good synthetic wig, it looks just as good as a wig made of human hair and is much cheaper.

For every day wear, be sure to buy cotton scarves; the silk ones slip off. Also, get long, rectangular ones because they're the easiest to work with. Buy as many colors and patterns as you can so you have lots of options when you're getting dressed.

It's helpful to get a few headbands too. Get the stretchy plain ones that are at the grocery or drug store. Wearing a headband makes it much easier to start the scarf tie because it not only anchors the scarf, but also gives the illusion of a hairline.

For those occasions when you just don't have time to play around with scarves, hats are perfect. Not just baseball caps, but fedoras, flouncy brims, cowboy hats, whatever. You have lots of options here. Try to keep as many choices as possible in your closet (or wherever), so that when it's time to get dressed, you can pick something that fits (or *makes*) your mood.

*

What should I do when my hair starts growing back?

Once you have a "shadow of hair" on your head, go to the salon and have them shave your neck so that the new growth on your head looks thick and groomed.

As your hair grows in, experiment with colors and shapes. I did. My stylist and I came up with lots of ideas together. She was really helpful.

She shaped a mohawk for me. Not like the spiky ones you see standing straight up on young people, but a stylish, subtle one with pastel coloring. It looked great. I never ever thought I would, but I can honestly say that I LOVE my short hair!

III. Surgery

"Time for you and time for me,
And time yet for a hundred indecisions,
And for a hundred visions and revisions,
Before the taking of a toast and tea."

– T.S. Eliot

I was faced with a decision about a mastectomy of only my right breast or a double mastectomy. To me, the thought of losing one or both of my breasts was terrifying. I had so many images in my head of women (in faraway countries) being brutalized in this way.

After much thought, I decided to go with symmetry and hopefully eliminate any worries of cancer showing up later in my left breast. I opted for a double mastectomy.

If you opt to have reconstructive surgery, your doctors will need to know before your mastectomy. Not an easy decision to make at that stage of your cancer journey, but it has to be done.

The reason is that during your mastectomy procedure, the surgeons place "expanders" in your chest wall under the pectoral muscle to plan for the reconstructive implants. The expanders are sacks (with valves) that can be filled with increasing amounts of saline over a period of weeks.

While I was contemplating whether to have reconstructive surgery, I was told that reconstruction after radiation (which was next for me in my treatment plan) was very difficult and would involve a complicated surgery.

> *Surgery decisions are so individual. Carefully review all of your options and then do what's right for YOU.*

Because of this information, I was actually leaning toward no reconstruction at all at the time. Having a flat chest didn't seem that daunting to me.

But then my plastic surgeon convinced me that if I decided to go for reconstruction, my particular surgery would be simpler than we had initially discussed. Cancer cells had not invaded my pectoral muscles, as we had originally feared. So I reconsidered and went ahead with the option of expanders under the pectoral muscles.

My plastic surgeon told me that I had a couple of other options: "back flap" or "tummy tuck" surgery. "Back flap" (also known as "latissimus") surgery is a process where your back muscle is threaded under your arm and around to your chest. A flap of skin is taken from your back to create a breast pocket for the implant.

I know. Sounds brutal. But the recovery time is actually quite minimal.

"Tummy tuck" (or TRAM flap) surgery uses muscle and fat from your abdomen to create a breast. No implant is required because fat from your tummy is used as filler. The recovery time for this type of surgery, I was told, is quite extensive.

> *Thoroughly read consent forms before signing anything. Make sure you aren't agreeing to a procedure that you and your medical team didn't already discuss.*

(An interesting side note about the "tummy tuck" surgery: You need a certain amount of fat to make it work. If you decide to gain weight for that purpose, be aware that any weight loss after surgery will shrink your breasts too, because the fat cells have no idea that they have been moved!)

*

I decided to go ahead with the simpler reconstructive procedure that used the pectoral muscle, even though I knew there was *some* risk because of the radiated tissue. My thinking was that the "back flap" and "tummy tuck" surgeries could be back-up options.

My plastic surgeon and breast cancer surgeon worked side-by-side during my operation. As my breast cancer surgeon performed the mastectomy, my plastic surgeon placed expanders under my pectoral muscle. During the same surgery, my breast cancer surgeon also removed and biopsied several lymph nodes to make sure they were cancer free.

After surgery, my plastic surgeon told me that both he and my breast cancer surgeon had been alarmed when they discovered that I had several hardened lymph nodes. He explained that hardened lymph nodes can sometimes be a sign that cancerous cells are still thriving and have not been treated effectively with chemo drugs. To compensate, my breast cancer surgeon removed thirty-two lymph nodes from my right armpit.

After I recovered from surgery, I went once a week for saline injections into my expanders. After each expansion, or "filling," it felt like there was an elephant standing on my chest. It was terribly uncomfortable, but the feeling only lasted for a day. After six weeks, I was finished with the expansion phase and was ready for radiation.

*

Where does the fluid from my surgery wound go?

After mastectomy surgery, I had a drain in my wound(s) to relieve some of the excess fluid and fiber that collects. The drains are tubes that have a clear bulb attached to the end to collect fluid.

> *Try to maintain a sense of humor. Even if a situation is only funny to you, laugh on the inside. It really does go a long way toward a healing body.*

I'll never forget . . .

I was in Walgreens shopping for headbands. I had the bulb part of my drain in my pants pocket, and the tubing was under my shirt, connecting my wound to the bulb.

I had finished my shopping and was headed to the checkout line when I noticed an older man walking towards me with a look of horror on his face. I looked down and realized that the bulb had popped out of my pants pocket and was dangling from the tubing that (I thought) was hidden under my shirt.

Yellow fluid had been leaking all over the store floor as I had been browsing from aisle to aisle. I was horrified! Embarrassed! Grossed out! All of the above! A memorable day!

*

Do all breast cancer patients get swollen arms?

Lymphedema (swollen arms) is a condition that causes enlarged, fluid-filled arms, often requiring the use of a pressure sleeve to keep the swelling under control. It's caused by the lack of lymph nodes in your armpits.

The job of lymph nodes is to filter and remove fluid from your body. When there aren't enough lymph nodes to do the job, the fluid doesn't know where to go, and it collects in your arm, causing it to swell.

Everyone's different, but the average number of lymph nodes under human armpits is forty. Lymph nodes are responsible for draining fluid from your arms and chest area. The more lymph nodes that are removed from your body (thirty-two in my case), the higher the risk of developing the dreaded lymphedema.

*

At this point in my treatment, my sense of humor was returning. A good sign. I was hopeful, but I still wasn't understanding why I continued to need radiation treatment if my cancerous nodes (all thirty-two of them!) had been removed during surgery. I asked my doctors, and they told me that treatment plans are based on the initial diagnosis and not on the outcome of previous treatments.

> *If you start to wonder about the timing of specific procedures as your treatment plan progresses, keep in mind that treatment plans are based on your initial diagnosis, not on the outcome of previous procedures.*

The reasoning behind the timing of my treatments (especially radiation) is something I wish I had understood from the beginning. Not that it would have changed anything; it just would have been nice to know.

IV. Radiation

"Remember the tea kettle – it is always up to its neck in hot water, yet it still sings."

- Author unknown

As I looked around the waiting room at my first radiation treatment appointment, I noticed there were people undergoing treatment for all kinds of problems, not just cancer. Some people had bulging tumors on their heads, faces, and necks – all pretty frightening!

Like me, most of the people were there for cancer. You could tell because they looked like they had just finished their chemo treatment and their hair was coming back.

Lots of "burr heads" all celebrating the little fuzz that was appearing. I'd never seen so many people talk so enthusiastically about their eyebrows and eyelashes!

*

What exactly happens during radiation treatments?

My particular radiation treatment was called "Intensity-Modulated Radiation Therapy." My treatments lasted about twenty minutes every weekday for six weeks.

When you check in for your appointment, you are identified by a computer imaging system that makes sure you are the right patient. You then go into a room that has a huge table with lots of knobs and adjustment handles on the side and a big satellite arm over it. The hard body mold that has been engineered for you is already in place to make sure that you stay in one position

The specifics of your treatment are prescribed by physicists, not your radiologist or oncologist.

during treatment.

Next you climb up and lie down on the table. The radiology technician makes sure that you are properly positioned on the table and then leaves the room. The clicking and whirring noises, rays of light, and flashes begin and continue to change angles and intensity for about twenty minutes.

My arms always went to sleep during treatments because they had to remain up over my head the entire time. It felt as though I was in a spaceship, watching all the gears and wheels slowly adjusting and moving to deliver their precise radiation rays. All very surreal.

*

What are the "negatives" of radiation?

Looking back, I never fully understood the damage to my lungs and other body tissue that the radiation rays would cause. At the time, I was more focused on applying topical creams to the affected areas of my skin so that they wouldn't blister and burn.

In hindsight, I wish I had realized the extent of the damage that the radiation treatments were inflicting on the rest of my body. Radiation basically causes scar tissue to form wherever tissue has been destroyed.

I doubt knowing the effects of radiation would have affected the end result; it just would have been nice to know—particularly the potential effects that it could have on my upcoming reconstructive procedure.

I used Eucerin Aquaphor (like a creamy version of Vaseline) to soothe my irritated skin.

V. Reconstruction

"Enjoy life sip by sip, not gulp by gulp."

– The Minister of Leaves

I was excited, optimistic, and ready to start my recovery. It had been one year and four months since my diagnosis. I reviewed the chronology of my cancer journey:

- Diagnosis *(February 2012)*
- Port Installation *(March 2012)*
- Chemotherapy *(March – July 2012)*
- Surgery for double mastectomy and expanders installation *(August 2012)*

- Daily radiation for six weeks
  (November – December 2012)

- Replace expanders with implants
  (April 2013)

I was so ready for getting back to "normal" and looking good! I checked into the surgical center for my reconstructive procedure, which involved replacing the expanders with implants. I had chosen smaller, tear-drop-shaped, silicone-filled implants. I was going for a more athletic-looking profile.

I had decided to also treat myself to a neck lift and dermabrasion around the mouth. The dermabrasion was the only thing that made me a little nervous because it looks like you've skidded across concrete on your face when you come out of surgery. But I was assured that it would heal quickly.

After surgery on Friday afternoon, I awoke from the anesthetic and felt goofy but good, and everyone was happy with the results. I went home that afternoon and slept away my weekend. I was on oral antibiotics as a precaution against infection.

By late Sunday evening, I started noticing that my right radiated breast area was very red and hot. Uh, okay. I'd been here before. I knew there was an infection brewing. I called my plastic surgeon the next morning and made an appointment. Sure enough, he was concerned.

Right away when he saw the infection, he said "damn radiation" and sent me off to an infectious disease specialist. The infectious disease doctor had the same sentiment about radiated tissue and its ability to attract whatever bacteria is floating around to help it flourish.

I was sent to the hospital to have a PICC line installed into my upper left arm. Another all-too-familiar procedure. I was then given intravenous antibiotics to be administered four times a day at home.

After two or three days of multiple daily infusions, I was getting worse, so I went back to the infectious disease doctor. He changed my antibiotic prescription to the strongest there was. But after two more days of daily infusions, my infection was even worse.

This was definitely not the way I had envisioned my reconstructive process!

It was now Friday again. A week had passed since my reconstructive surgery and I was back in my surgeon's office to figure out what to do next. I knew what was coming. My surgeon told me that my reconstructive surgery was not working out as he'd hoped and that my right breast implant had to be removed to get over the infection. His thinking was that removing the foreign implant would clear everything up.

So exactly one week after my first reconstructive surgery, I was back under general anesthesia to have my right breast implant removed.

> *Intravenous (IV) antibiotics can worsen any depression you might be already enduring.*

I was SO disappointed about my failed reconstruction. I was beginning to feel so discouraged and depressed. Very unlike me.

I must say though that my left breast is quite beautiful and without complications. My right breast, not so much!

*

When I came home from implant removal surgery, I had a PICC line in my arm and the dreaded drain (like the one I'd had after my mastectomy). I looked at the area that had previously been my red, inflamed right breast and burst into tears. What was left was a scooped-out dent with weird extra skin around it. It looked as if an amateur had been practicing making balloon animals with my skin.

So much for my vision of symmetry, which was one of the reasons I had opted for a double mastectomy in the first place.

In the beginning of this journey of mine, I had worried about symmetry and the appearance of reconstructed breasts. But that was no longer even on my radar. I just wanted to be rid of the infection.

Various intravenous (IV) antibiotics were administered through my PICC line, and astonishingly, the infection raged on. It had been almost four weeks since my original reconstructive surgery and I was being scheduled for yet another surgery to "clean things out." My doctor said that this time he was going to open the incision and remove all of the radiated tissue.

> *As you go from treatment to treatment and doctor to doctor, try to get as many "side effect" questions answered as you can. The information you learn might not necessarily affect the outcome of the treatment, but it will make you feel less crazy.*

So again I went under anesthesia and hoped for the best. After surgery, I was sent home from the hospital with instructions to change the gauze bandages twice daily and apply ointment to the affected areas.

The first time I changed the bandage, I was horrified. I had three open slashes on my chest.

I called my doctor's nurse and told her that the doctor had forgotten to close the wound! She assured me that was the way it was supposed to be so that the wounds could heal from the inside out, preventing any closed pockets of infection from occurring. Good to know!

*

It turns out that the radiation was the culprit of my persistent infection and failed reconstruction. There was a lot of dead tissue inside my wound from my radiation treatment and my body was trying to get rid of it.

Radiation is, apparently, the foe of many plastic surgeons. Who knew? There are many plastic surgeons who will not even attempt to operate on body tissue that has been radiated. Another thing I hadn't realized about radiation is that not only are its effects cumulative, but they continue to build for years.

> *Don't forget that radiation rays affect cancer cells AND other parts of your body.*

*

Are post-cancer treatment pills considered chemotherapy?

While spending time in and out of various hospitals as my doctors tried to heal my infection, I was repeatedly asked the same questions about my health history. One of the questions was: "Are you still on chemo?"

I always responded by saying, "No, my last chemo infusions were completed ten months ago, and my last Herceptin infusion was two months ago. Now I am just on estrogen blockers for ten years."

That was my understanding and my standard response.

Well, it turns out I was wrong. In the first hospital where I stayed for my infection treatments, an oncology nurse was assigned to give me the estrogen blocker that I had been taking on my own every morning at home. She did *not* treat it like a routine task.

In the second hospital I stayed in, again an oncology nurse was assigned to give me my pill. This time not only was my pill in a plastic bottle, but it had also been placed in a sealed plastic baggy.

The nurse had to put on two pairs of rubber gloves before she opened the pill bottle. Then she carefully dropped the pill directly on my tongue.

She discarded the gloves that she had used by wrapping them around the pill bottle and the baggies. She then carefully disposed of it all in a nearby HazMat container.

So, yes, I guess I *am* on chemo now, in the form of estrogen blockers, and will be for the next ten years. And apparently, what I take every morning as part of my routine scares everyone who is in charge of delivering it to me!

*

What's next?

It has been a very long year and a half. I recently developed lymphedema in my right arm and hand and am searching for a solution. The solution could be a massage, acupuncture, something else, or all of the above.

I wear a compression sleeve at night, and during the day I sometimes wrap my arm to control the swelling. It aches and hurts, but it won't kill me.

I have a very knowledgeable and compassionate oncology rehabilitation specialist. Her name is Julia Osborne. She's helping me with my lymphedema. She has become a great friend and sounding board and has helped me discover my "new normal."

Life *does* go on. With excellent days and sad days and days in between. Every day is now brilliantly intense and real-time and means another day of winning this battle and feeling stronger and more determined.

I came across a quote that I would like to share because it sums up my new outlook on life and living.

"Life just doesn't care about our aspirations or sadness. It's often random, and it's often stupid and it's often completely unexpected and the closures and the epiphanies and revelations we end up receiving from life, begrudgingly, rarely turn out to be the ones we thought (we'd have)."

- *Khaled Hosseini, author*

Your cancer experience will change you profoundly. Try to consider it a tremendous learning experience; a golden opportunity to clarify life's priorities.

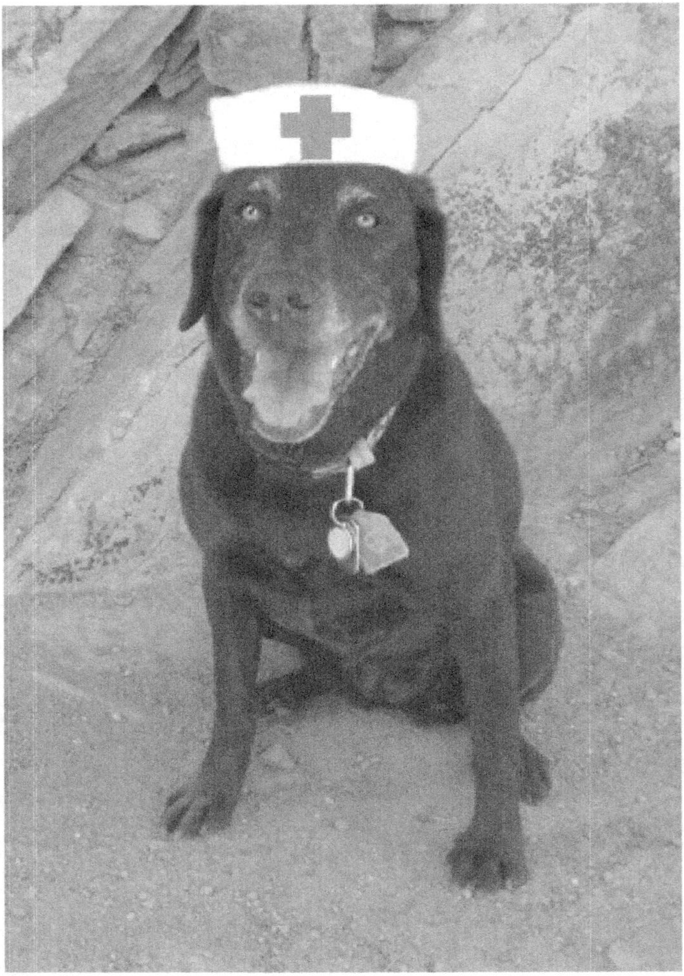

"Nurse Chloe"

Acknowledgements

Perhaps the magnitude of this disease should be gauged by the number of players on the team.

I would like to thank all of my dedicated doctors who have been integral to my recovery. My breast imaging radiologist who diagnosed me, Therese Kaske, MD, my kind and caring oncologist, Robin Kovachy, MD, my upbeat and intelligent breast cancer surgeon, Jane Kercher, MD, my awesome plastic surgeon, Gary Snider, MD, my kind and brilliant IMRT radiologist, Seth Reiner, MD, and my infectious disease doctors, Ray Blum, MD and Josephine Williams, MD.

My heartfelt gratitude to Dr. Rachel Norwood, without whose support and wisdom I could not have made this journey. And to Julia Osborne, my oncology rehab specialist, who has been a lifesaver in treating the lymphedema that followed my surgery.

My deep gratitude to my friend, Trish Thorpe, who was willing to take on the task of turning my random, meandering journal into an organized book that I hope provides helpful information for those on similar odysseys.

And, of course, my husband, Larry, my daughter, Karen, my grandsons, Hayden and Carson, and my son, Chris, and his wife, Michelle, who were sources of constant support and cheerleading.

To order this book from Amazon:

http://www.amazon.com/Trish-Thorpe/e/B009AF8OJ0/ref=ntt_athr_dp_pel_1

Made in the USA
Monee, IL
05 November 2026

67352871R00062